ISBN: 1469923734
ISBN-13: 978-1469923734

I0429675

"CARE OF YOUR BABY'S TEETH"

(A Parental Guide to Caries Free Dentition in Children)

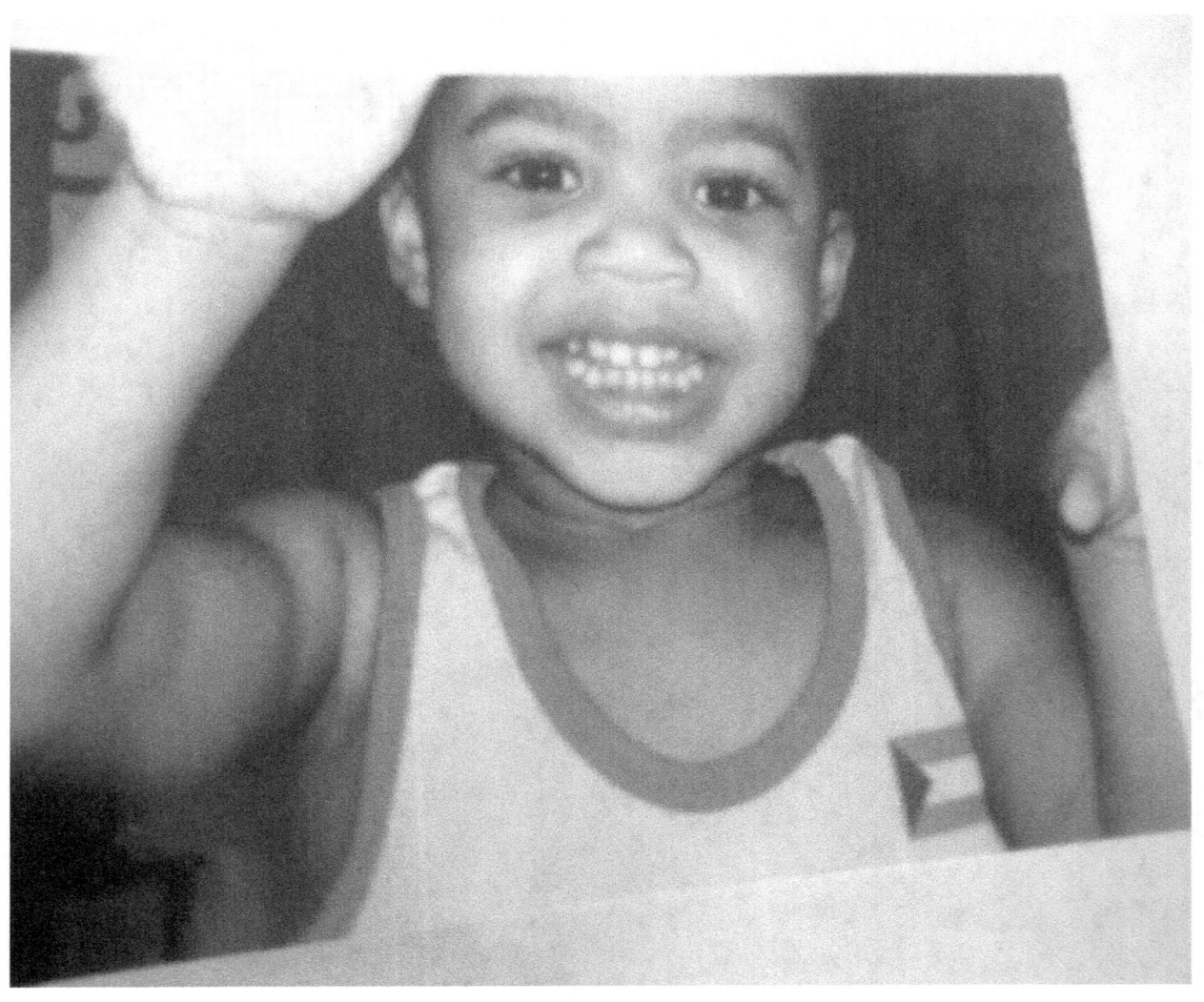

Dr. Emmanuel W. Francis D.D.S.

Dedication

I dedicate this book to my wife, Andrea, who has successfully raised our children – Ishmael, Denise, and Kendra, free of dental caries, and look forward to the day when all Bahamian mothers can do the same.

PREFACE

The high incidence of nursing bottle caries in young children in the Bahamas is alarming. A significant number of parents and guardians seem to be unaware of factors that cause tooth decay in early childhood, and are contributing directly to this problem by putting babies to bed with bottles in the mouth. I have preached about this problem to parents who present with children suffering from this disease with little decrease in its occurrence nationally after about 30 years.

Moreover, many parents do not know much about teeth, nor about the importance of healthy baby teeth to their child's overall health. Baby teeth (primary teeth) can best be described as foundation teeth, since they pave the way for the permanent teeth (secondary teeth). It is also a misconception that these primary teeth can be discarded without consequence, since they would be replaced by permanent ones; but children need their teeth to eat properly at any age.

Primary school age children have a mixed dentition of primary and permanent teeth. Neglect of the teeth at this age not only causes destruction of the baby teeth but simultaneously destroys the first permanent molars which begin to erupt at about age 6 years.

Dental disease processes and their causes are discussed in this book. With this information, preventative measures which could be implemented by parents and guardians to stop these maladies from occurring are presented. The essential role of the dental health care provider in all of this is also explained.

It is hoped that this guide will be the start of a new era in dental education in the Bahamas, and be used by child caretakers and educators alike to raise the dental I.Q. of all who read it. Our children can then look forward to healthy, happier lives free of dental

diseases under the guidance of well informed parents and guardians.

TABLE OF CONTENTS

Chapter 1

What You Should Know About Baby Teeth

There are twenty (20) teeth in the primary dentition called baby teeth. Ten (10) are in the upper jaw or maxilla, and ten (10) are in the lower jaw or mandible. All teeth have crowns, which you see in the mouth, and roots that you do not see which are anchored in bone.

(i) <u>**Types of Teeth (See Diagram #1)**</u>

<u>**The following represents the number of teeth in each jaw:**</u>

(A) Front (Anterior) Teeth – Central Incisors (2), Lateral Incisors (2) Cuspids or Canines (2)

(B) Back (Posterior) Teeth – First molars (2) Second Molars (2)

Diagram # 1

Types of Primary Teeth

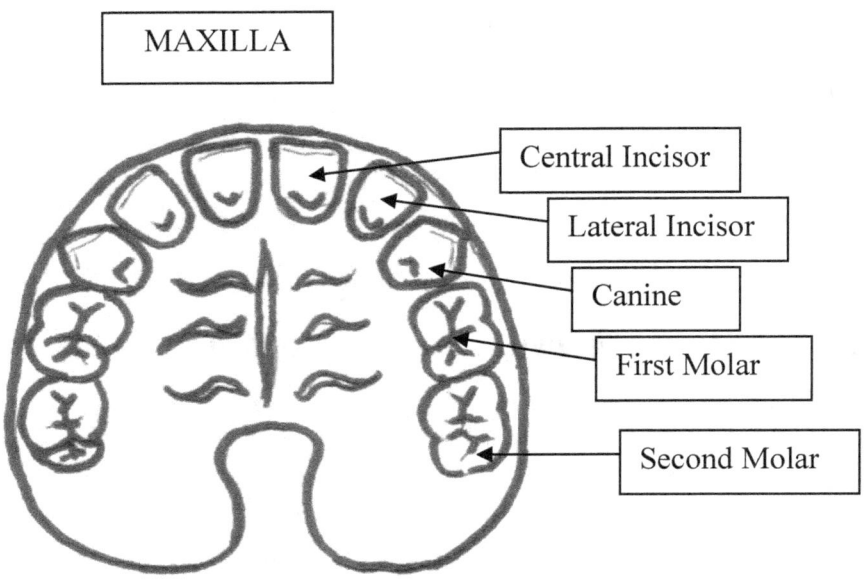

MAXILLA

Central Incisor

Lateral Incisor

Canine

First Molar

Second Molar

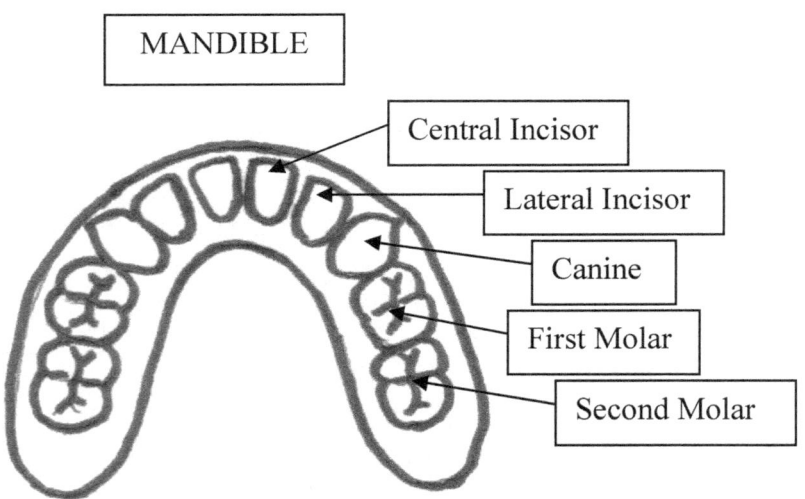

MANDIBLE

Central Incisor

Lateral Incisor

Canine

First Molar

Second Molar

Anatomy of Teeth (See Diagram #2)

Teeth are made up of four (4) tissues. These are enamel, dentin, pulp and cementum. The pulp is the soft tissue that provides blood and nerve supply to the tooth. The bulk of the tooth is dentin with enamel covering the crown (the part you see in the mouth), and cermentum covering the root.

(ii) **Anatomy of the Supporting Tissues (See Diagram #2)**

(A) Alveolar Bone – Bony "process" of the jaws that provides the house or socket which holds the teeth in place.

(B) Periodontal Ligament – connective tissue that binds the teeth to the alveolar bone by attaching to the root cementum.

(C) Gingiva (gums) – tough (keratinized) soft tissue that covers the alveolar bone and attaches to the teeth like a collar at the base of the crown (neck of the tooth).

Diagram # 2
Anatomy of Teeth and Supporting Tissues
(Longitudinal Section)

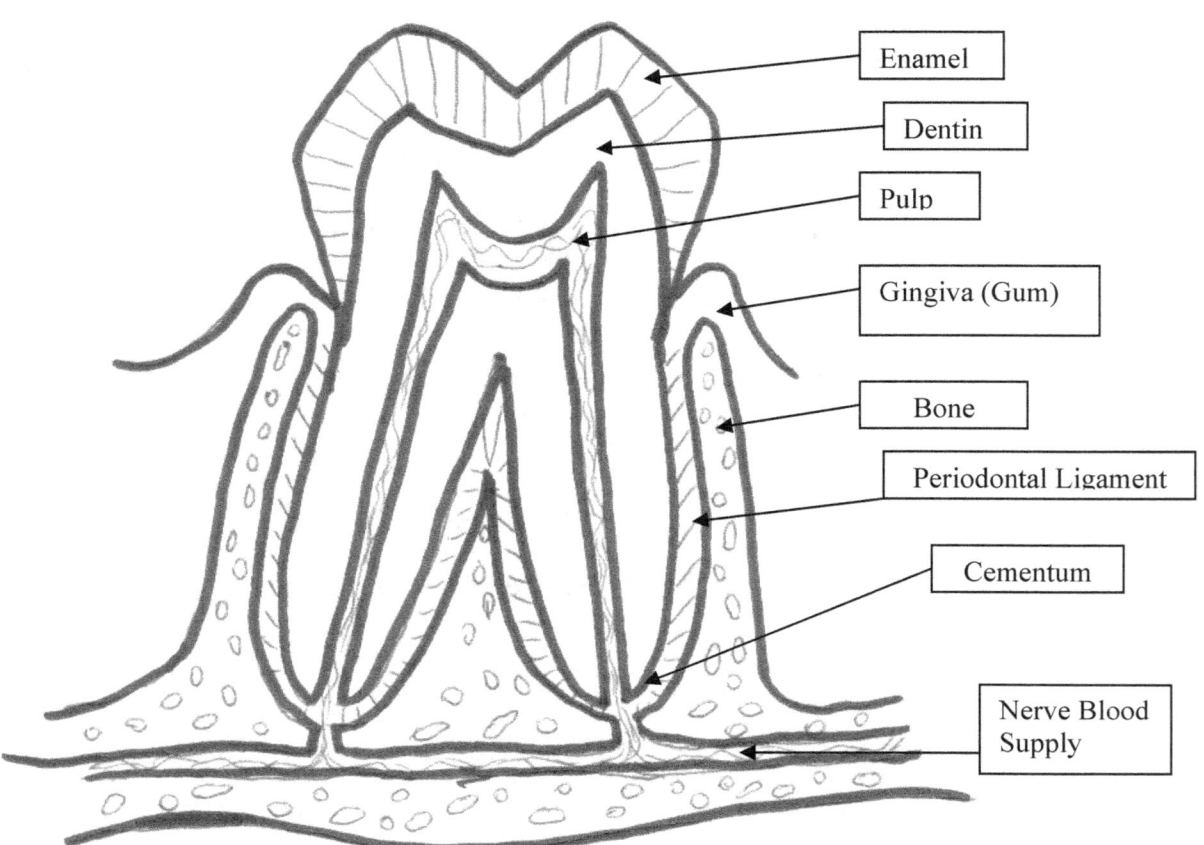

Enamel

Dentin

Pulp

Gingiva (Gum)

Bone

Periodontal Ligament

Cementum

Nerve Blood Supply

(iii) <u>**Eruption of teeth (Cutting Teeth)**</u> – Baby teeth begin to erupt at about age six (6) months starting with the lower central incisors. In successive months, the eruption pattern continues with the upper centrals, lower laterals, upper laterals, lower canines, upper canines, lower first molars, upper first molars, lower second molars, and finally upper second molars. By about age two (2), all the primary are in place but their roots may not fully form until about age three (3). This is the ideal time for the child's first dental visit.

At about age six (6) years, the baby teeth start to change in the order that they erupt. The permanent incisors erupt behind the primary ones and are pushed into position by action of the tongue, after the baby teeth are shed (exfoliate). Sometimes the permanent front teeth are larger than the space left behind by the baby teeth that they replace. When this occurs, adjacent primary teeth need to be extracted to allow the permanent ones to be pushed into proper alignment by the tongue.

It is very important to know that the first permanent molars come in behind the primary teeth about the same time that the permanent centrals erupt. The lower teeth usually come in ahead of the uppers. These are the permanent teeth that are affected when the baby teeth are neglected, and are often the first permanent teeth needing fillings or extractions (pulling). Care is taken by dental health care providers to protect these with sealants (protective covering) soon after they erupt.

Chapter 2

Development of Teeth

Baby teeth begin to form about four (4) months in utero (womb). The enamel forms first, is about 99% mineral and is the hardest tissue in the body. It is at this stage that fluoride, if present, is incorporated into the enamel crystal to form fluoroapatite, which is harder and more resistant to decay than the normal hydroxyapatite crystals of enamel. Too much fluoride, when ingested, will cause the enamel to be discolored and mottled as seen in some of the southern Bahamian islands where fluoride concentration in well water is high.

Formation of the dentin and pulp follows. The crown, which forms first, is complete in bone and erupts (is pushed out) by growth of the root. Eruption pain (teething pain) is expected due to inflammation of the gingival tissue (gums), which may be accompanied by infection from bacteria. Your dentist may prescribe analgesics (pain killers) and antibiotics (infection medication) in severe cases of teething pain.

Development of the teeth is possible because of adequate blood supply from dental arteries, veins and nerves that innervate the pulp through an opening at the tip of the root called the apical foramen. If blood supply to the tooth is cut off (e.g. traumatic injury), development would cease and pulp death will follow. When this happens, the tooth will gradually become darker and develop abscess (gum boil).

Proper nutrition is essential to the development of all oral (mouth) tissues, and indeed, the whole body as well. Nutritional deficiencies e.g. lack of minerals, vitamins, essential proteins and fats can adversely affect the development of teeth, bone and gums.

Developmental disturbances of enamel and dentin in children can be caused by infection, trauma, lead poisoning, radiation treatment for cancers, excessive dietary fluoride, Rubella (German Measles) during pregnancy, brain injury, nerve defects, allergic reactions and some medications, e.g., tetracycline, which intrinsically (inside) stains the teeth when taken during teeth development.

Genetic disorders also affect development. The most significant are dentinogenesis imperfecta and emelogenesis imperfecta, which are hereditary conditions that adversely affect the development of these tissues (dentin and enamel). Micrognathia is also a congenital (inherited) condition resulting in undersized mandible which creates special problems with feeding.

Cleft lip and cleft palate are developmental anomalies (not normal) affecting children and present challenges with feeding and esthetics (looks). These defects have to be corrected surgically and should not be left untreated.

Chapter 3

Dental Disease Processes and Nursing Bottle Caries

There are two types of dental disease processes: (i) Tooth decay (caries) (ii) Periodontal disease ("gum disease").

(i) **Dental Caries**

This disease is an infectious process caused by bacterial that live in the mouth. The main causative organism is streptococcus mutans, a bacterium which is introduced to the mouth from parents and others by exchange of saliva from intimate kissing, or by sharing spoons and other feeding utensils with the child. These bacteria feed primarily on fermentable carbohydrates (sugars – including lactose, the sugar present in milk). The bacterial fermentation of the sugars produce acid, which removes mineral (leaching) from the enamel, thus weakening it. This demineralization of the enamel can be reversed by brushing the teeth and allowing minerals from the saliva to migrate back into the enamel. Brushing is essential to caries prevention because it removes bacterial plaque off the teeth.

The constant exposure of teeth to milk, juices or any liquid that contains sugar (e.g. sleeping with the bottle) does not allow remineralization to take place and promotes the growth of acidic bacterial plaque in layers. Eventually the enamel dissolves and is lost forever exposing the softer, darker dentin to attack. Dentin is affected by acids as well as bacterial digestion of its organic components causing pain, poor feeding habits and abscesses. When this happens in bottle feeders it is called "nursing bottle caries". Bottle use should be stopped at about age 2 years.

Unfortunately, many decayed teeth must be extracted (pulled) by a dentist resulting in premature loss of the foundation teeth (baby teeth), which are necessary for eating and the proper alignment of permanent teeth which develop under them.

Dental caries can be restored with silver amalgam or composite resin fillings when the decay does not reach the pulp. Baby teeth with infected pulp could also be saved by pulp therapy, i.e., pulpotomy, followed by stainless steel crown restorations, if abscess formation has not occurred.

(ii) **Periodontal Disease:**

Bacterial plaque is the cause of periodontal disease, and is an invisible sticky film that forms on the teeth in less than eighth (8) hours. If this plaque is not removed, e.g. brushing and flossing, it builds up in layers and becomes discolored by pigments in colored foods and beverages. Eventually, minerals from the saliva migrate into the plaque and causes it to calcify (harden), forming what is called calculus (tartar).

This bacterial deposit affects the supporting tissues of the teeth with irritants that cause inflammation and infection of the gums, periodontal ligament and alveolar bone. In the early stages, inflammation of the gums develops with swelling, redness, pain and bleeding (gingivitis). This inflammation spreads to deeper tissues where infection sets in, resulting in bone loss, discharge of pus, (pyorrhea) and pocket formation between the teeth and bone (periodontitis). Unchecked periodontal disease results in tooth loss by loosening of the attachment and destruction of the bony socket. It also causes halitosis (bad breath), pain, bleeding, drifting of teeth and periodontal abscesses. Periodontal disease is more prevalent in adults as it usually takes years to develop, but can manifest in some children who are at risk due to diet, lifestyle (oral hygiene), crooked teeth or juvenile diabetes.

Chapter 4

Preventive Dentistry – Oral Hygiene, Prophylaxis (Cleaning), Fluoride Treatment and Sealants

Oral Hygiene:

Oral hygiene is the best method used to prevent dental caries and periodontal disease. The main objective (goal) is the removal of bacterial plaque from the teeth, gums, tongue and hard palate (roof of the mouth). This can be effectively done through regular brushing with a soft or medium bristle brush; American Dental Association approved toothpaste, and flossing.

Younger children need assistance with brushing and flossing, especially before bedtime. A soft, clean wash cloth could also be useful in infants for effective oral hygiene. Proper method for brushing and flossing should be taught by your dentist or dental hygienist. Children should be supervised to ensure that they do not eat the toothpaste as this could cause excessive intake of fluoride.

Prophylaxis (cleaning of teeth or prophy)

The dental hygienist is the health care provider who is especially trained in oral examinations, oral hygiene instruction, cleanings, fluoride treatment, placement of sealants and dental radiography (X-rays). This dental health auxiliary was introduced to reduce the workload on the dentist who also does these treatments.

Effective cleaning is achieved by removing all tartar (calculus, plaque and stains) from the teeth. This process is called scaling as deposits come off like scales off a fish when it is cleaned. Polishing of the teeth follows with a rotary (spinning) brush or rubber cup and prophy paste. Flossing completes the cleaning process.

Dental cleanings should not be painful. Any discomfort during the procedure should be noted to avoid repetition. It is extremely important to avoid the association of dental treatment with pain, especially with cleanings, because we want to encourage our patients, at an early age, to seek regular cleanings.

Fluoride Treatment:

After prophylaxis, topical fluoride gels may be applied to arch shaped, trays and placed in contact with teeth for about four (4) minutes. This process allows for fluoride ions to be incorporated into the surface of the enamel, creating teeth more resistant to tooth decay. This must be done by a trained professional to prevent toxicity from ingestion of fluoride. After the treatment is completed, rinsing, eating or drinking is to be avoided for at least thirty (30) minutes, to maximize to topical effect. Topical applications should be repeated every six (6) months and must always be preceded by a proper prophylaxis (cleaning).

Public health initiatives have promoted mass topical fluoridation through fluoride oral rinse programs in public schools.

Sealants:

Sealants are viscous (thick) liquid resins that harden when mixed with a catalyst, or when ultraviolet light is shined on them. They are placed on molar teeth in children to seal pits and fissures (clefts) on the occlusal (biting) surfaces. This makes them more resistant to pit and fissure cavities, which are the most common type of cavities.

It is important to note that sealants are placed to prevent caries in permanent teeth and should not be used to "seal" pits and fissures one cavities have formed. These teeth should be fiilled properly, which requires complete removal of decay.

Chapter 5
Nutrition and Dental Health

Proper nutrition is important in the growth and development of healthy teeth, bone and guns. Similarly, a healthy mouth is necessary to enjoy a proper diet. Since teeth and bone begin forming in the womb, it is important for the expecting mother to practice proper nutrition. The dentist should be informed about the patient's pregnancy during consultation to ensure safe treatment choices and to allow him/her the opportunity to give appropriate nutritional advice.

Good nutrition can best be achieved by eating a variety of foods. Diets that are restrictive and limited to only a few preferred items will no doubt fall short of some nutrients. The best dietary regimen should consist of a balance of proteins (meat, eggs, poultry, fish, beans, etc.), carbohydrates (breads, cereals, rice, grits, pasta, etc.), fruits (oranges, apples, pears, peaches, peppers, bananas, grapefruits, mangoes etc.), vegetables (corn, carrots, beets, cabbage, lettuce, potato, onion, broccoli, squash, cauliflower, etc.) and dairy (milk, cheese, yogurt, butter, etc.).

Raw, fresh foods are generally better, but some like meats, beans, potatoes, rice and grits are best cooked. Raw fruits and vegetables are considered "detergent" foods because they scrub plaque off the teeth during mastication (chewing), and is " God's way" of natural cleansing for the teeth. Moreover, the chewing of these "hard" foods scrubs the gums free of plaque and also makes them tougher. Medically, plant based foods are high in fiber which promotes a healthy gut and regular bowel movement.

Vitamins and minerals are necessary nutrients and are best obtained through eating a balanced diet. Supplements may be used to ensure adequate intake of these nutrients, but care must be taken not to exceed the recommended does of vitamins A, D, E, K (fat soluble vitamins), which become toxic when taken in excess. During pregnancy, it is necessary to ensure that vitamins and minerals are present as nutrients. Vitamins A, D, and C along with minerals calcium, magnesium and phosphorus are essential to the formation of teeth and bone. A, C, and B – complex vitamins ensure healthy gums and soft tissue. Fluoride concentration of one part per million (1.p.p.m) in drinking water is believed to promote caries resistant enamel when taken during enamel formation.

In these modern times, refined foods are common and a lot of them contain sugars. As was discussed earlier, sugar consumption is directly related to both tooth decay and gum disease. It is therefore important to read labels on these processed food items for information on nutrient content and added sugars. Sugars may be disguised as high fructose corn syrup, maltodextrin sucrose, honey, dextrose, mannitol, fructose, etc..

Unfortunately, many cold cereal preparations have too much added sugar, which is why children who are accustomed to sweets crave them. Even if cereals are manufactured without sugar, children who like sweets will add their own sugar when they mix them with milk. I strongly recommend that parents and guardians ensure that unnecessary sugars are eliminated from their child's diet at birth, starting with bottle feeding of milk and juices. Parents must be aware that sugar has been proven to be addictive, like heroin and cocaine, and cravings can be uncontrollable and harmful to other parts of the body as well.

Water is essential and is the best beverage on earth. It is needed for all body functions, and is ideal for washing sugars off the teeth when the toothbrush is not available. Sodas should be excluded from the diet or mixed with water to dilute their high sugar content. One twelve-ounce (12 oz.) container of soda may have many as twelve (12) or more teaspoons of sugar in it. Raw, fresh fruits and nuts are good substitutes for highly refined, processed sweets when snacks are desired. Never put sodas in a baby's bottle; it will literally melt their teeth if left in long enough.

C. Everette Koop (The Former U.S. Surgeon General) noted: "Your choice of diet can influence your long term health prospects more than any other action you might take." I always ask the question: "If sugar can damage your teeth that you can see, what do think it will do to the parts of your body that you can't see?"

Conclusion

Early childhood dental disease is preventable and can be eradicated by utilization of the dental knowledge contained in this book. A healthy, happy and more enjoyable life awaits children whose parents are educated about the causes of dental disease, and are willing to make the necessary life style changes that ensure good dental health in their offspring.

Moreover, the burden of the cost of health care for children can be greatly reduced for both parents and governmental social services alike.

The prophet Hosea once wrote: "My people are destroyed for a lack of knowledge". If you reject knowledge, your children will be the ones that will suffer. Train them well in dental disease prevention and when they become old they will not depart from it.

References

1. McDonald, R , Avery, D, B (1978) " Dentistry for the Child and Adolescent" (Third Edition).

2. Nigel, A, E, (1981) "Nutrition in Preventive Dentistry"

3. Avena, N.M., Rada, P., & Hoebel, B.G. (2008) Evidence of Sugar Addiction: Behavioral and neurochemical effects of intermittent, excessive sugar intake. Neuroscience & Behavioral Reviews, 32(1), 20-39.

4. Francis, R (2002) "Never Be Sick Again: Health is a Choice, Learn How to Choose It". Florida: Health Communications Inc.

5. Desjardins,N (2010). The Sugar Free Lifestyle: 7 Day Sugar Free Diet. eBook Guides 4 Liife.com

Index